BLOOD GLUCOSE REVOLUTION

A Revolutionary Approach to Managing Your Blood Glucose Level

BY

Max Hunter

TABLE OF CONTENT

PREVENTION AND DELAY OF COMPLICATIONS
OVERALL WELL-BEING AND QUALITY OF LIFE

CONCLUSION

INTRODUCTION

Living with imbalanced blood glucose levels can be a daunting experience. Whether you are dealing with diabetes or simply striving for optimal health, understanding and effectively managing your blood glucose is crucial. The traditional methods of monitoring and controlling blood sugar may have served you well, but what if there's an even better way?

In this book, we will explore a revolutionary approach to managing blood glucose levels. It is a paradigm shift that takes into account not only the food we eat but also the impact of lifestyle factors, emotions, stress, and more. We will uncover the interconnectedness of these elements and how they influence your blood glucose levels.

The Blood Glucose Revolution empowers you to take control of your health and well-being. It offers a comprehensive understanding of the underlying mechanisms that affect blood glucose and provides practical strategies to achieve balance. Our goal is not

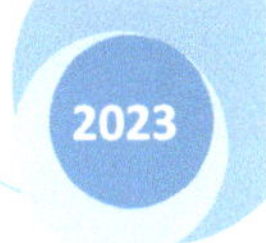

just to stabilize blood sugar, but to revolutionize your approach to managing it.

Throughout this ebook, we will delve into cutting-edge research, share real-life success stories, and present actionable steps you can implement in your daily life. Whether you are a newly diagnosed diabetic, a health-conscious individual, or a healthcare professional seeking fresh insights, this book will provide valuable knowledge and tools to support your journey.

It's time to break free from the limitations of old beliefs and embrace a new era of blood glucose management. Get ready to embark on a transformative journey and unlock the secrets of the Blood Glucose Revolution. Together, let's pave the way towards optimal health and well-being.

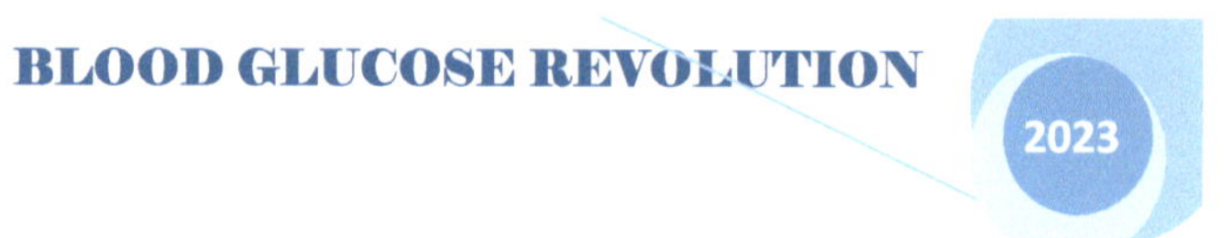

CHAPTER ONE

Understanding Blood Glucose

In this chapter, we will delve into the fundamental concepts of blood glucose and its significance in managing diabetes. Understanding how blood glucose levels work and what factors can affect them is essential for adopting the revolutionary approach to managing blood glucose effectively.

WHAT IS BLOOD GLUCOSE?

Blood glucose, also known as blood sugar, refers to the amount of glucose present in the bloodstream. Glucose is the primary source of energy for our bodies and plays a crucial role in various bodily functions. When we consume carbohydrates, our bodies break them down into glucose, which is then transported through the bloodstream to provide energy to cells.

THE IMPORTANCE OF BLOOD GLUCOSE CONTROL

Maintaining blood glucose within a healthy range is essential for overall health and well-being, especially for individuals with diabetes. High or low blood glucose levels can lead to various health complications and symptoms. Consistently high blood glucose levels (hyperglycemia) can damage blood vessels, nerves, and organs over time, while low blood glucose levels (hypoglycemia) can result in dizziness, confusion, and even loss of consciousness.

BLOOD GLUCOSE TESTING

Regular monitoring of blood glucose levels is a critical component of managing diabetes. Testing blood glucose levels provides valuable information about how the body is responding to food, medication, physical activity, and other factors. Blood glucose testing can be done using a glucose meter, which measures the glucose concentration in a small blood sample obtained from a finger prick or alternate testing sites.

NORMAL BLOOD GLUCOSE LEVELS

Normal blood glucose levels vary depending on the timing of the test. Fasting blood glucose levels, measured after at least 8 hours of fasting, should ideally be between 70 and 100 mg/dL (3.9-5.5 mmol/L). Postprandial blood glucose levels, measured 1-2 hours after a meal, should generally be below 180 mg/dL (10 mmol/L).

FACTORS AFFECTING BLOOD GLUCOSE LEVELS

Several factors can influence blood glucose levels, including:

• **Diet:** The types and amounts of carbohydrates, proteins, and fats consumed can affect blood glucose levels.

• **Physical Activity**: Exercise and physical activity can lower blood glucose levels by increasing glucose uptake by muscles.

• **Medications:** Certain medications, such as insulin and oral hypoglycemic agents, can directly impact blood glucose levels.

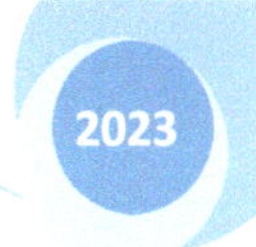

- **Stress:** Emotional or physical stress can cause blood glucose levels to rise.
- **Illness:** Infections, fevers, and other illnesses can cause blood glucose levels to fluctuate.

Understanding these factors and their effects on blood glucose levels will help you make informed decisions and take appropriate actions to manage your blood glucose effectively.

CHAPTER TWO

The Traditional Approach to Managing Blood Glucose

In this chapter, we will explore the traditional methods and strategies that have been commonly used to manage blood glucose levels. While these approaches have been effective for many individuals, the revolutionary approach takes a more comprehensive and holistic perspective that we will discuss in later chapters.

1. Medication and Insulin Therapy

The traditional approach to managing blood glucose often involves the use of medication or insulin therapy. Medications such as metformin, sulfonylureas, or DPP-4 inhibitors are commonly prescribed for individuals with type 2 diabetes to help regulate blood glucose levels. For individuals with type 1 diabetes or advanced type 2 diabetes, insulin injections or an insulin pump may be necessary to supplement the body's insulin production.

2. Blood Glucose Monitoring

Regular blood glucose monitoring is a crucial component of the traditional approach. By testing blood glucose levels using a glucose meter, individuals can track their levels and make necessary adjustments to medication, diet, or physical activity. Self-monitoring of blood glucose (SMBG) allows individuals to identify patterns, understand how different factors impact blood glucose levels, and make informed decisions.

3. Meal Planning and Carbohydrate Counting

Meal planning is a common practice in the traditional approach to managing blood glucose. It involves carefully selecting foods, controlling portion sizes, and monitoring carbohydrate intake. Carbohydrate counting is a technique used to estimate the amount of carbohydrates in a meal and adjust insulin doses accordingly. This approach helps individuals maintain stable blood glucose levels by balancing insulin doses with carbohydrate intake.

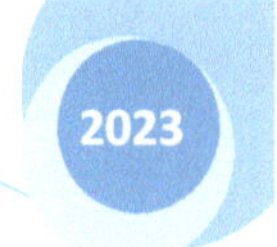

4. Physical Activity

Physical activity is often recommended as part of the traditional approach to managing blood glucose. Exercise can help improve insulin sensitivity, lower blood glucose levels, and enhance overall health. Regular aerobic exercise, strength training, and other forms of physical activity can be beneficial in managing blood glucose and reducing the risk of complications.

5. Healthcare Provider Support

In the traditional approach, individuals typically work closely with healthcare providers, including doctors, nurses, dietitians, and diabetes educators. These professionals provide guidance, prescribe medications, and offer education on blood glucose management techniques. Regular check-ups and consultations help individuals stay on track and make any necessary adjustments to their treatment plans.

BLOOD GLUCOSE REVOLUTION

CHAPTER THREE

The Revolutionary Approach to Managing Blood

GLUCOSE LEVELS

In this chapter, we will explore the revolutionary approach to managing blood glucose levels. This approach takes a fresh perspective on blood glucose management, focusing on a holistic and individualized approach that goes beyond traditional methods. By understanding the underlying principles and implementing this approach, individuals can achieve better control over their blood glucose levels and experience improved overall health and well-being.

1. Holistic Approach

The revolutionary approach recognizes that blood glucose management is not just about the food we eat or the medications we take. It considers the interconnectedness of various factors, including nutrition, physical activity, stress management, sleep, and

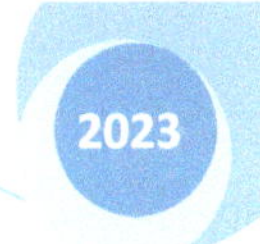

emotional well-being. By addressing all these aspects together, individuals can achieve optimal blood glucose control.

2. Individualization

Each person's body is unique, and their response to different interventions can vary. The revolutionary approach emphasizes the importance of individualization in blood glucose management. It encourages individuals to understand their own body's response to different foods, exercise routines, and lifestyle factors. By personalizing their approach, individuals can find what works best for them and make informed decisions about their blood glucose management.

3. Carbohydrate Awareness

Carbohydrate intake has a significant impact on blood glucose levels. The revolutionary approach focuses on carbohydrate awareness, emphasizing the quality and quantity of carbohydrates consumed. It encourages individuals to choose complex carbohydrates with a low glycemic index and to monitor portion sizes.

By understanding how different carbohydrates affect their blood glucose, individuals can make informed choices and maintain better control.

4. Mindful Eating

Mindful eating is a core component of the revolutionary approach. It involves paying attention to hunger and satiety cues, eating slowly, and savoring each bite. By practicing mindful eating, individuals can develop a healthier relationship with food, avoid overeating, and make conscious choices that support stable blood glucose levels.

5. Physical Activity

Regular physical activity plays a crucial role in blood glucose management. The revolutionary approach promotes incorporating physical activity into daily routines, emphasizing both aerobic exercise and strength training. Exercise helps improve insulin sensitivity, promotes weight management, and contributes to overall cardiovascular health. By finding enjoyable activities and incorporating them into their lifestyle, individuals can reap the benefits of regular exercise for blood glucose control.

6. Stress Management

Chronic stress can have a negative impact on blood glucose levels. The revolutionary approach recognizes the importance of stress management techniques such as meditation, deep breathing exercises, and engaging in activities that promote relaxation. By managing stress effectively, individuals can minimize the impact of stress hormones on blood glucose levels and improve overall glycemic control.

7. Sleep Optimization

Sufficient and quality sleep is essential for maintaining stable blood glucose levels. The revolutionary approach emphasizes the importance of prioritizing sleep hygiene and developing healthy sleep habits. By getting an adequate amount of sleep each night, individuals can support optimal blood glucose regulation and improve their overall health.

8. Continuous Glucose Monitoring (CGM)

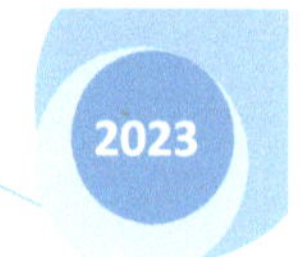

The revolutionary approach embraces technological advancements, such as continuous glucose monitoring (CGM). CGM devices provide real-time information about blood glucose levels, allowing individuals to make immediate adjustments to their diet, exercise, or medication if necessary. CGM empowers individuals to have a deeper understanding of their blood glucose patterns and facilitates more effective management.

By adopting this revolutionary approach to blood glucose management, individuals can take control of their health and achieve better blood glucose control. The holistic and individualized nature of this approach promotes overall well-being and provides a foundation for long-term success in managing blood glucose levels.

CHAPTER FOUR

Implementing the Revolutionary Approach

In this chapter, we will provide a step-by-step guide to adopting the revolutionary approach to managing blood

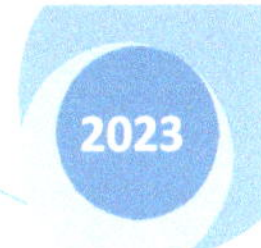

glucose levels. We will explore dietary changes, meal planning, and the importance of physical activity and exercise in maintaining stable blood glucose levels. By following these practical steps, individuals can integrate the principles of the revolutionary approach into their daily lives.

1. Assess Your Current Diet

Start by evaluating your current diet and identifying areas that may need improvement. Look for foods high in refined carbohydrates, added sugars, and unhealthy fats. Take note of portion sizes and the frequency of meals and snacks throughout the day.

2. Embrace Whole, Unprocessed Foods

The revolutionary approach emphasizes the importance of whole, unprocessed foods. Increase your intake of fruits, vegetables, whole grains, lean proteins, and healthy fats. These nutrient-dense foods provide essential vitamins, minerals, and fiber while promoting stable blood glucose levels.

3. Monitor Carbohydrate Intake

Pay close attention to the carbohydrates you consume. Choose complex carbohydrates with a low glycemic index, such as whole grains, legumes, and non-starchy vegetables. Be mindful of portion sizes and distribute your carbohydrate intake evenly throughout the day to avoid spikes in blood glucose levels.

4. Practice Mindful Eating

Adopting mindful eating habits can positively impact blood glucose control. Slow down during meals, chew your food thoroughly, and savor each bite. Listen to your body's hunger and fullness cues, stopping when you feel comfortably satisfied. This approach can prevent overeating and support stable blood glucose levels.

5. Meal Planning and Prepping

Plan your meals to ensure a well-balanced and blood glucose-friendly diet. Include a variety of nutrients in each meal, such as lean proteins, whole grains, healthy fats, and plenty of non-starchy vegetables. Prepare and portion your meals ahead of time to make healthier choices easily accessible throughout the week.

6. Consider Glycemic Load

Alongside monitoring carbohydrates, also consider the glycemic load of your meals. The glycemic load takes into account both the quality and quantity of carbohydrates consumed. It provides a more accurate measure of how a particular food or meal affects blood glucose levels. Aim for meals with a moderate glycemic load to promote stable blood glucose control.

7. Engage in Regular Physical Activity

Physical activity plays a crucial role in managing blood glucose levels. Incorporate both aerobic exercise and strength training into your routine. Aim for at least 150 minutes of moderate-intensity aerobic activity per week, along with two or more days of strength training exercises. Consult with your healthcare provider before starting any new exercise program.

8. Find Activities You Enjoy

To maintain long-term adherence to physical activity, choose activities that you enjoy. Whether it's walking, dancing, cycling, swimming, or playing a sport, find

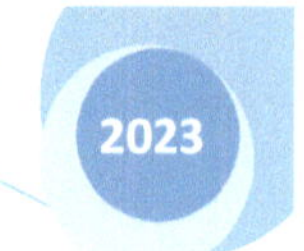

something that brings you joy and fits your lifestyle. Incorporate activities into your daily routine, such as taking the stairs instead of the elevator or going for a walk during your lunch break.

9. Monitor Your Blood Glucose

Regularly monitor your blood glucose levels to assess the impact of dietary changes and physical activity. Use a blood glucose meter or consider utilizing a continuous glucose monitoring (CGM) system for real-time feedback. Adjust your diet, exercise, and medication based on your blood glucose readings, and consult with your healthcare provider for guidance.

10. Seek Professional Support

If needed, consult with a registered dietitian or certified diabetes educator for personalized guidance and support. They can help tailor dietary recommendations, provide meal planning assistance, and offer strategies for managing blood glucose levels effectively.

By following this step-by-step guide, individuals can adopt the revolutionary approach to managing blood glucose levels successfully. Incorporating dietary

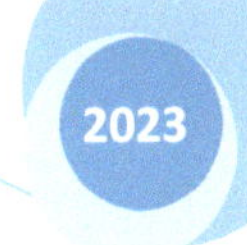

changes, meal planning, and regular physical activity will provide a strong foundation for stable blood glucose control and improved overall health. Remember, progress takes time, so be patient with yourself and celebrate each small step towards better blood glucose management.

CHAPTER FIVE

Monitoring and Tracking Blood Glucose

In this chapter, we will explore the importance of monitoring and tracking blood glucose levels as part of the revolutionary approach to managing blood glucose. We will discuss various monitoring techniques, introduce continuous glucose monitoring (CGM), and provide tips for interpreting and analyzing blood glucose data. By actively monitoring and tracking blood glucose, individuals can make informed decisions and adjust their approach to achieve optimal control.

IMPORTANCE OF BLOOD GLUCOSE MONITORING

Regular blood glucose monitoring is a crucial aspect of managing blood glucose levels effectively. It provides valuable information about how your body responds to different foods, medications, physical activity, and other lifestyle factors. Monitoring allows you to identify

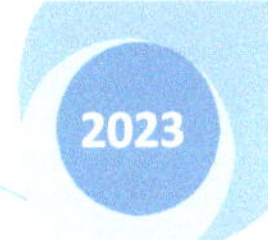

patterns, make necessary adjustments, and maintain stable blood glucose levels.

SELF-MONITORING OF BLOOD GLUCOSE (SMBG)

Self-monitoring of blood glucose involves using a glucose meter to measure your blood glucose levels at home. Follow these tips for effective SMBG:

- **Establish a routine:** Set a schedule for monitoring your blood glucose. Consistency is key to capturing meaningful data and identifying patterns.

- **Proper technique:** Familiarize yourself with the instructions for using your glucose meter. Ensure you have clean hands, use a lancet to obtain a small blood sample, and follow the meter's specific guidelines.

- **Record your results:** Keep a record of your blood glucose readings along with additional relevant information, such as the time of day, medication or insulin doses, meals, physical activity, and any notable factors that may influence your readings.

- **Review and analyze:** Regularly review your blood glucose records to identify trends, patterns, and any potential factors affecting your readings. Look for patterns related to specific meals, exercise routines, or medication adjustments.

CONTINUOUS GLUCOSE MONITORING (CGM)

Continuous glucose monitoring (CGM) is an advanced method of blood glucose monitoring that provides real-time information about your glucose levels throughout the day. CGM involves wearing a sensor that measures glucose levels under the skin, and transmitting data to a receiver or smartphone app. Consider these aspects when using CGM:

- **Accuracy and calibration:** Follow the calibration instructions provided by the manufacturer to ensure accurate readings. Regularly calibrate your CGM device as recommended to maintain accuracy.

- **Data interpretation:** Utilize the CGM data to track your glucose levels continuously. Identify trends,

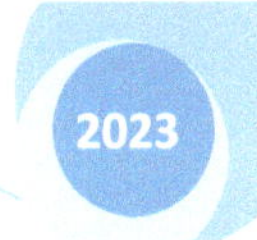

patterns, and glucose excursions to gain insights into how your body responds to different factors.

- **Real-time feedback:** Take advantage of the real-time alerts and alarms provided by CGM devices. These notifications can help you make immediate adjustments to your diet, physical activity, or medication as needed.

- **Collaborate with healthcare providers:** Share your CGM data with your healthcare team during appointments. They can help analyze the data, make informed recommendations, and guide your blood glucose management.

PATTERN MANAGEMENT

Monitoring blood glucose levels allows you to identify patterns that may impact your management. Look for patterns related to specific meals, exercise routines, stress levels, or medication adjustments. Once you identify patterns, you can make targeted changes to your diet, activity levels, or medications to address them and maintain stable blood glucose control.

DATA TRACKING AND ANALYSIS

Use digital tools, apps, or spreadsheets to track and analyze your blood glucose data effectively. These tools can help visualize trends, calculate averages, and provide a comprehensive overview of your blood glucose management. Regularly review your data and make adjustments to your approach as needed.

COLLABORATE WITH HEALTHCARE TEAM

Share your blood glucose records, whether obtained through SMBG or CGM, with your healthcare team. They can provide valuable insights, interpret the data, and help you make informed decisions. Collaborating with your healthcare provider allows for personalized guidance and adjustments to your management plan.

Remember, blood glucose monitoring is not just about the numbers; it's about gaining insights into your body's response and making informed decisions. Regular monitoring and tracking will empower you to make necessary adjustments, optimize your approach, and achieve better blood glucose control as part of the revolutionary approach.

CHAPTER SIX

Overcoming Challenges and Obstacles

Managing blood glucose levels can indeed present challenges, but with the right strategies and mindset, they can be overcome. In this chapter, we will address common barriers and obstacles that individuals face in managing their blood glucose levels. We will provide practical strategies and tips for overcoming these challenges and maintaining long-term success.

EMOTIONAL AND PSYCHOLOGICAL CHALLENGES

Managing blood glucose levels can be emotionally and psychologically demanding. Here are some strategies to overcome these challenges:

• **Education and Support:** Seek out resources, support groups, or educational programs that provide information and guidance on blood glucose management. Connecting

 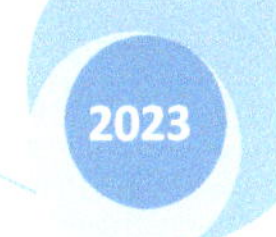

with others who face similar challenges can be empowering and reassuring.

- **Mindfulness and Stress Reduction:** Engage in stress-reducing activities such as meditation, deep breathing exercises, or hobbies that bring you joy. Managing stress can positively impact blood glucose control.

- **Mental Health Support:** If you are struggling with emotional challenges, anxiety, or depression related to your blood glucose management, consider seeking professional help from a therapist or counselor who specializes in chronic illness or diabetes management.

LIFESTYLE ADJUSTMENTS

Making lifestyle adjustments to manage blood glucose levels may require changes in routines and habits. Here's how to navigate these adjustments:

- **Gradual Changes:** Implement changes gradually, allowing yourself time to adjust and adapt. This approach makes it more sustainable and manageable in the long run.

- **Set Realistic Goals:** Set achievable goals that align with your capabilities and lifestyle. Break them down into smaller steps to track progress and maintain motivation.

- **Plan and Prepare:** Incorporate meal planning, physical activity schedule, and organization techniques into your routine. This will help you stay on track and reduce the chances of making impulsive choices that may impact blood glucose levels.

SOCIAL SITUATIONS AND PEER PRESSURE

Managing blood glucose levels can be challenging in social situations. Here's how to handle these situations effectively:

- **Communication:** Educate your friends, family, and loved ones about your blood glucose management needs. Explain why certain choices are important to you and seek their support and understanding.

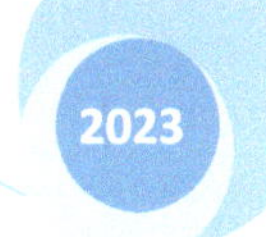

- **Plan Ahead:** Before attending social events, communicate with the host or restaurant staff about your dietary needs. Offer to bring a dish that aligns with your blood glucose goals. Planning ahead can help you navigate the available options more effectively.

- **Assertiveness:** Be assertive and confident in advocating for your health needs. Politely decline offerings that may disrupt your blood glucose control and instead focus on healthier alternatives.

PLATEAUS AND SETBACKS

Sometimes, despite your best efforts, you may experience plateaus or setbacks in blood glucose management. Here's how to navigate these situations:

- **Persistence and Patience:** Understand that blood glucose management is a lifelong journey with ups and downs. Stay committed to your goals, be patient with yourself, and don't let setbacks discourage you.

- **Seek Professional Guidance:** If you're facing persistent challenges or are unsure about the best course of action, consult with your healthcare provider or diabetes educator. They can provide individualized guidance and support.

- **Learn from Setbacks:** Use setbacks as learning opportunities. Reflect on what may have contributed to the setback and explore strategies to prevent similar situations in the future.

Remember, managing blood glucose levels is a continuous process, and it's natural to encounter challenges along the way. By being proactive, seeking support, and adopting a resilient mindset, you can overcome these obstacles and maintain steady progress in your blood glucose management journey as part of the revolutionary approach.

CHAPTER SEVEN

Long-Term Benefits of the Revolutionary Approach

The revolutionary approach to managing blood glucose levels offers numerous long-term benefits that extend

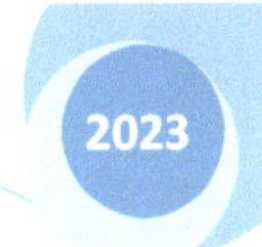

beyond immediate glycemic control. In this chapter, we will explore the significant advantages individuals can experience by adopting this approach as a sustainable lifestyle. From improved overall health to enhanced quality of life, the long-term benefits are transformative.

OPTIMAL BLOOD GLUCOSE CONTROL

The primary objective of the revolutionary approach is to achieve and maintain optimal blood glucose control. By implementing the principles outlined in this approach, individuals can experience stable blood glucose levels within the target range. This reduces the risk of acute complications and long-term complications associated with diabetes, such as cardiovascular disease, kidney problems, and nerve damage.

ENHANCED ENERGY LEVELS

Balancing blood glucose levels through the revolutionary approach promotes stable energy levels throughout the day. By avoiding sharp spikes and crashes in blood glucose, individuals can experience sustained energy, improved concentration, and increased productivity.

Stable energy levels enable individuals to engage in activities they enjoy and fulfill their daily responsibilities with vitality.

WEIGHT MANAGEMENT

The revolutionary approach focuses on nutrition, mindful eating, and portion control. By making healthier food choices and maintaining a balanced diet, individuals can achieve and maintain a healthy body weight. Weight management is essential in blood glucose control, as excess body weight can lead to insulin resistance and hinder glycemic control. Achieving a healthy weight reduces the risk of obesity-related complications and improves overall well-being.

CARDIOVASCULAR HEALTH

The revolutionary approach promotes heart-healthy choices, such as consuming nutrient-dense foods, engaging in regular physical activity, and managing stress. By adopting these habits, individuals can improve their cardiovascular health and reduce the risk of heart disease, high blood pressure, and other related

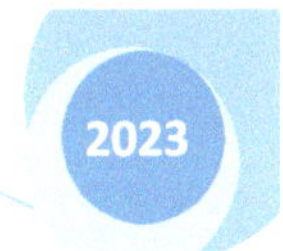

conditions. Maintaining optimal blood glucose levels further protects the heart and blood vessels, contributing to long-term cardiovascular well-being.

REDUCED MEDICATION DEPENDENCY

The revolutionary approach empowers individuals to take control of their blood glucose levels through lifestyle modifications. By optimizing nutrition, physical activity, and overall health, individuals may experience a reduction in medication requirements. This is particularly relevant for individuals with type 2 diabetes, as lifestyle changes can often result in improved glycemic control and decreased reliance on medication. However, any changes in medication should be made in consultation with a healthcare professional.

IMPROVED MENTAL HEALTH

The revolutionary approach acknowledges the importance of mental and emotional well-being in blood glucose management. By adopting stress management techniques, practicing mindfulness, and seeking support, individuals can experience improved mental health.

Balanced blood glucose levels also contribute to stable moods and enhanced overall psychological well-being.

PREVENTION AND DELAY OF COMPLICATIONS

Maintaining optimal blood glucose control through the revolutionary approach reduces the risk of complications associated with diabetes. By managing blood glucose levels within the target range, individuals can prevent or delay the onset of complications such as diabetic retinopathy, neuropathy, nephropathy, and cardiovascular disease. This allows for a higher quality of life and minimizes the impact of diabetes-related complications.

OVERALL WELL-BEING AND QUALITY OF LIFE

By implementing the revolutionary approach, individuals can enjoy an overall improved sense of well-being and enhanced quality of life. Stable blood glucose levels, increased energy, reduced medication dependency, and better physical and mental health contribute to a greater ability to engage in daily activities, pursue personal goals, and enjoy life to the fullest.

It's important to note that the long-term benefits of the revolutionary approach are cumulative and dependent on consistent adherence to the principles outlined. Each individual's experience may vary, and it's crucial to consult with healthcare professionals for personalized guidance and support. By embracing this approach and making it a sustainable lifestyle, individuals can achieve significant long-term benefits and thrive in their blood glucose management journey.

CONCLUSION

In the revolutionary approach to managing blood glucose levels, we have explored a comprehensive and holistic approach that goes beyond simply controlling numbers on a glucose meter. This approach focuses on making sustainable lifestyle changes, including dietary modifications, meal planning, regular physical activity, and emotional well-being.

By adopting this approach, individuals can experience a wide range of benefits. These include improved blood glucose control, enhanced energy levels, weight management, better cardiovascular health, reduced medication dependency, improved mental health, prevention and delay of complications, and an overall improved quality of life.

While there may be challenges along the way, such as emotional hurdles, lifestyle adjustments, social situations, and plateaus, we have provided strategies and

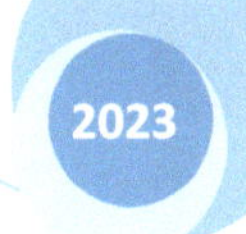

tips for overcoming these obstacles. By staying persistent, seeking support, and maintaining a resilient mindset, individuals can navigate these challenges and continue their journey toward optimal blood glucose control.

Additionally, we have addressed frequently asked questions to provide clarity and guidance on various aspects of the revolutionary approach. It is important to remember that personalized advice from healthcare professionals is essential to tailor the approach to individual needs and circumstances.

By embracing the revolutionary approach and making it a part of your daily life, you have the power to take control of your blood glucose levels and improve your overall well-being. Stay motivated, celebrate your progress, and remember that small steps can lead to significant long-term benefits. You have the ability to revolutionize your blood glucose management and live a healthier, more fulfilling life.

www.ingramcontent.com/pod-product-compliance
Lightning Source LLC
Chambersburg PA
CBHW040309240726
48664CB00006B/1433